28 Daily Somatic Exercises for Weight Loss: Enhance Flexibility, Strength, and Balance for Physical and Emotional Well-Being through Daily Routines.

ANGEL ROSIE

TABLE OF CONTENTS

Introduction

In our contemporary pursuit of well-being, the concept of somatics has emerged as a beacon of holistic health. But what exactly are somatic exercises? At its essence, somatics is an approach that recognizes the inseparable link between the mind and the body. It's a philosophy that transcends the mere physicality of exercise, delving into the realms of awareness, perception, and conscious movement.

Somatic exercises are not just about burning calories or sculpting muscles; they're about fostering a deep understanding of one's own body. Through intentional, mindful movements, these exercises aim to release chronic muscular tension, improve mobility, and, in the context of our exploration, contribute to a healthier weight. This isn't a quick fix or a one-size-fits-all solution; it's a journey inward, where you'll discover the potential for change resides within your very being.

The Mind-Body Connection in Weight Loss:

The age-old adage "mind over matter" takes on a new dimension when we consider weight loss through the lens of the mind-body connection. Weight management is often reduced to diet plans, calorie counting, and vigorous workouts, neglecting the powerful influence of our mental and emotional states on our physical well-being.

In this introduction, let's dismantle the notion that weight loss is solely about external transformations. Instead, we'll explore the intricate interplay between our thoughts, emotions, and bodily responses. Through somatic exercises, we aim to tap into the body's innate wisdom, aligning our mental and physical selves to achieve sustainable, long-term weight loss.

As I guide you through the chapters ahead, envision a shift in perspective. Picture weight loss not as a battle against your body but as a collaborative journey where your mind and body work in harmony. This book is not just a guide to shedding pounds; it's an invitation to a profound exploration of self – an exploration that transcends the superficial and embraces the transformative power of embodied awareness.

So, buckle up for a unique odyssey. Together, we'll navigate the terrain of somatic exercises, unveiling their potential to redefine your relationship with your body and reshape your understanding of weight loss.

As we venture into the core principles of somatics and its application in weight management, I encourage you to approach each concept with an open mind and a willingness to engage with the exercises on a deeper level. This is not a race; it's a journey. And like any meaningful journey, it begins with a single step – a step into the realm of somatic solutions for holistic weight loss.

Chapter one

Understanding Somatics

Embarking on a journey of somatic exercises is akin to setting sail on uncharted waters. Before we dive into the intricacies of these transformative movements, let's illuminate the compass guiding our exploration—understanding somatics. In this section, we unravel the tapestry of somatic principles, revealing a philosophy that transcends the conventional boundaries of physical fitness.

Definition and Principles of Somatics:

At its core, somatics is an invitation to become intimately acquainted with the language of our own bodies. It is both a philosophy and a practice that recognizes the interconnectedness of our physical, emotional, and mental states. Somatic exercises engage us in a process of self-discovery, inviting us to listen to the whispers of our bodies and respond with conscious, intentional movement.

The principles of somatics are grounded in the belief that the body holds the key to its own healing and well-being. Unlike traditional exercise routines that may focus solely on external performance, somatic exercises prioritise internal awareness. This inward focus allows us to identify and release habitual patterns of muscular tension, ultimately restoring a sense of balance and ease in our movements.

As we delve into somatics, we encounter the concept of sensory-motor amnesia—a term coined by Thomas Hanna, a pioneer in the field. This phenomenon refers to the body's tendency to forget how to release certain muscles voluntarily due to chronic stress or repetitive movements. Somatic exercises aim to reverse this amnesia, guiding us back to the innate intelligence of our bodies and enabling us to reclaim lost ranges of motion.

How Somatic Exercises Differ from Traditional Workouts:

To grasp the essence of somatic exercises, it's essential to discern their divergence from conventional workouts. While traditional approaches often emphasise external exertion and performance, somatics prioritises internal sensing and awareness. It's not about pushing the body to its limits but rather about understanding and cooperating with its inherent wisdom.

In a somatic practice, movements are deliberate, slow, and mindful. Each exercise becomes an opportunity for exploration, a dialogue with the body's signals. This contrasts sharply with the high-intensity, rapid-paced routines that dominate many fitness regimens. Somatic exercises invite us to cultivate a relationship with our bodies, fostering a sense of trust and cooperation.

Furthermore, somatics challenges the prevailing mindset that views the body as a machine to be trained and mastered. Instead, it encourages us to perceive the body as a living, dynamic entity capable of continuous self-regulation and healing. By embracing this perspective, we shift from an external locus of control to an internal one, empowering ourselves to participate actively in our well-being.

Benefits of Integrating Somatics into Weight Loss Programs:

As we navigate the landscape of weight loss, it's crucial to recognize the unique benefits that somatic exercises bring to the table. Beyond the conventional methods of diet and rigorous workouts, somatics introduces a nuanced approach—one that addresses the root causes of weight-related challenges.

Somatics and Stress Reduction:

Chronic stress is a formidable adversary in the battle against excess weight. Somatic exercises act as allies in stress reduction, promoting relaxation through intentional movements and breathwork. By engaging the relaxation response, we mitigate the impact of stress hormones on the body, fostering an environment conducive to healthy weight management.

Enhanced Body Awareness:

The journey toward weight loss is often hindered by mindless, habitual behaviours. Somatic exercises elevate our body awareness, unveiling the unconscious patterns that may contribute to weight gain. Through this heightened awareness, we gain the tools to make informed choices, fostering a more mindful relationship with food and movement.

Improved Posture and Alignment:

The way we carry ourselves influences not only our physical well-being but also our perception of self. Somatic exercises target muscular imbalances and postural misalignments, promoting a balanced and aligned body. This not only enhances our physical presence but also contributes to the efficiency of our movements, laying a foundation for sustainable weight loss.

Efficient Movement Patterns:

In the realm of somatics, movement is not solely about burning calories; it's about moving with efficiency and grace. By reprogramming inefficient movement patterns, somatic exercises optimise the body's functionality. This efficiency extends beyond the exercise mat, influencing our daily activities and contributing to a more active, energised lifestyle.

In the chapters that follow, we will delve deeper into these principles and explore specific somatic exercises tailored to support your weight loss journey. But before we embark on the practical aspects, let this understanding of somatics serve as a compass, guiding us through the uncharted waters of holistic well-being and mindful weight management.

Chapter two

Embodied Awareness

Embarking on the exploration of embodied awareness is akin to stepping into a sanctuary of self-discovery, where the boundaries between mind and body blur, and the whispers of our physical being beckon us into a profound journey. In this section, we'll navigate the intricate landscape of embodied awareness, understanding how it serves as the cornerstone of somatic exercises and, by extension, mindful weight loss.

Cultivating Mindful Eating Habits:

The journey of weight loss often begins on our plates, yet the act of eating is frequently shrouded in distraction. In the realm of embodied awareness, we uncover the transformative power of mindful eating—a practice that extends far beyond the mere consumption of food.

Mindful eating invites us to engage all our senses in the dining experience. It's about savouring each bite, appreciating the textures and flavours, and acknowledging the nourishment that food provides. As we cultivate this awareness, we begin to discern the subtle cues of hunger and satiety, liberating ourselves from the confines of external diets and calorie counts.

Picture a moment of mindful eating: the vibrant colours of a salad, the aroma of freshly prepared meals, the textures dancing on your taste buds. In this state of heightened awareness, food becomes more than fuel; it becomes a source of connection and joy. Through somatic practices, we rekindle our relationship with food, transforming it from a battleground to a realm of mindful nourishment.

Tuning into Hunger and Fullness Cues:

Our bodies communicate with us in a language of sensations, a symphony of cues that guide us in maintaining a harmonious relationship with food. Yet, amidst the noise of modern life, we often find ourselves out of tune with these signals. Embodied awareness directs our attention inward, allowing us to tune into the subtle messages of hunger and fullness.

Consider the simple act of having a meal. How often do we eat out of habit, boredom, or stress, ignoring the signals of our body? Embarking on the path of embodied awareness involves relearning to listen. Somatic exercises provide a canvas for this reconnection, helping us discern authentic hunger from emotional cravings and honouring the body's cues for nourishment.

By cultivating awareness around our eating habits, we not only foster a healthier relationship with food but also lay a foundation for weight loss rooted in balance. It's not about rigid dietary rules but about tuning into the body's wisdom, allowing it to guide us toward nourishment that is both satisfying and aligned with our well-being.

The Role of Body Awareness in Weight Management:

As we navigate the labyrinth of weight management, body awareness emerges as our guiding light. It's the compass that steers us away from external dictates and toward an intuitive understanding of our bodies. In the context of somatic exercises, body awareness is not a passive observation but an active engagement—a dialogue with the physical self.

Imagine standing before a mirror, not to critique imperfections but to marvel at the intricate dance of muscles and bones that carry you through life. This shift in perception, from criticism to appreciation, is the essence of body awareness. Through somatic practices, we learn to inhabit our bodies fully, embracing their uniqueness and acknowledging the wisdom they hold.

Body awareness extends beyond the exercise mat, influencing our posture, movements, and daily choices. It's the foundation upon which we build a sustainable approach to weight management. By fostering a conscious connection with our bodies, we become attuned to their needs, responding with kindness and respect rather than judgement and restriction.

In the chapters that follow, we will delve into specific somatic exercises designed to deepen embodied awareness. These exercises are not mere physical motions; they are invitations to be present in each moment, to savour the richness of our bodily experiences, and to forge a path toward mindful weight loss.

As we continue this journey, let the practice of embodied awareness be a lantern guiding you through the intricate passages of self-discovery. Embrace the whispers of your body, for in their subtle messages lies the roadmap to a healthier, more harmonious relationship with both yourself and the journey toward holistic well-being.

Chapter three

Core Somatic Exercises

As we venture into the realm of somatic exercises, we arrive at a cornerstone of mindful movement—the exploration of our core. In this section, we will delve into the intricacies of core somatic exercises, unravelling the transformative potential they hold for not just sculpting abdominal muscles but fostering a profound connection between our physical and mental selves.

Gentle Body Movements for Core Activation:

The core, often associated with washboard abs and superficial aesthetics, is, in essence, the epicentre of our physical being. Beyond the allure of a toned midsection, the core serves as the nexus for stability, strength, and the harmonious integration of movements. Somatic exercises designed to activate the core go beyond traditional crunches and sit-ups, inviting us into a world of gentle yet powerful body movements.

Let's consider a foundational somatic exercise for core activation: the pelvic tilt. This simple movement involves tilting the pelvis forward and backward while lying on your back. As you engage in this gentle rocking motion, you tune into the sensations around your lower abdomen and spine. Notice the subtle engagement of muscles, the release of tension, and the way your breath naturally synchronises with the movement.

The key here is not to perform the movement mechanically but to engage in a dialogue with your body. Picture it as a conversation where you're attentively listening to the feedback—each tilt becomes a sentence, and the sensations are the words that guide you. Through these deliberate, mindful movements, you awaken the core muscles, fostering a connection that goes beyond the superficial layer of aesthetics.

Breathing Techniques for Abdominal Engagement:

Breath, the constant companion to our movements, is often overlooked in traditional fitness practices. In the realm of somatics, the breath takes centre stage as a facilitator of core engagement. Through specific breathing techniques, we harness the power of the diaphragm and cultivate a dynamic interplay between breath and movement.

Consider the diaphragmatic breath—a foundational technique in core somatic exercises. As you inhale, allow your abdomen to expand like a balloon, feeling the breath fill the lower lungs. Then, on the exhale, envision a gentle contraction of the abdominal muscles, guiding the breath out. This conscious coordination of breath and abdominal engagement transforms a simple act into a profound somatic exercise.

Now, integrate this breathwork into a familiar movement, such as a seated twist. As you inhale, lengthen through the spine, and as you exhale, engage the core to facilitate the twist. The breath becomes a guiding force, a rhythm that orchestrates the movement and ensures a harmonious interaction between the respiratory and muscular systems.

Somatic Yoga Poses for Core Strength:

Yoga, with its ancient roots in holistic well-being, seamlessly intertwines with somatic principles to offer a treasure trove of poses that cultivate core strength. In the realm of somatic yoga, the focus is not on achieving contorted postures but on moving with awareness and intention, allowing the body to unfold at its own pace.

Consider the Cat-Cow pose, a staple in many yoga sequences. In the somatic approach, this classic duo becomes more than a warm-up—it becomes an exploration of the core. As you move into the arching (cow) and rounding (cat) of the spine, each transition becomes an opportunity to sense the engagement of core muscles. It's not about how far you can stretch; it's about the quality of movement and the depth of connection with your core.

Extend this exploration to a seated posture, such as Boat Pose (Navasana). In somatic yoga, this pose becomes a canvas for refining the quality of engagement. Rather than forcefully lifting the legs, the focus is on initiating the movement from the core, feeling the subtle activation of abdominal muscles supporting the legs' elevation. Through this intentional approach, core strength becomes an integrated aspect of the entire body, rather than an isolated achievement.

Examples of Core Somatic Exercises:

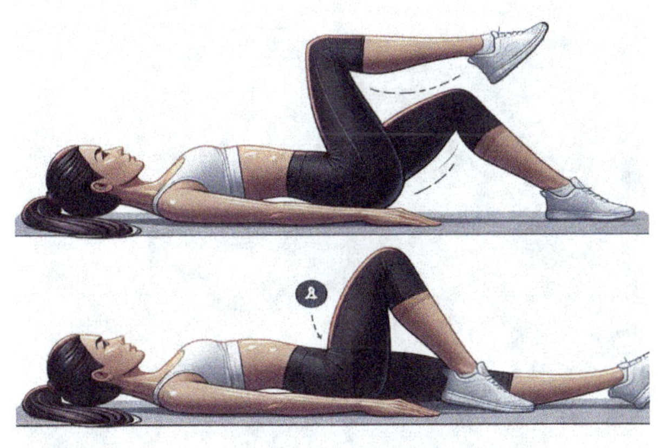

Pelvic Tilt:
- Lie on your back with knees bent and feet flat on the floor.
- Inhale and gently tilt your pelvis upward, arching your lower back.

- Exhale and tilt your pelvis downward, flattening your lower back against the floor.
- Repeat this rocking motion, paying attention to the sensations in your lower abdomen and lower back.

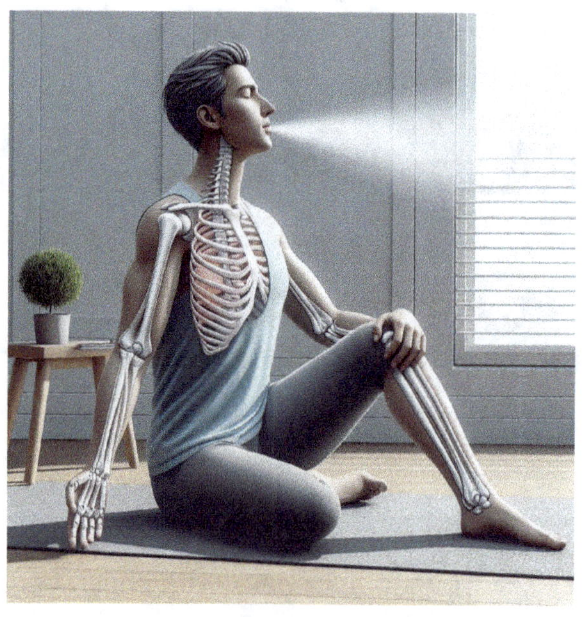

Diaphragmatic Breath in Seated Twist:
- Sit comfortably with a straight spine.

- Inhale deeply, allowing your abdomen to expand.
- Exhale slowly, engaging your core as you twist to one side.
- Inhale back to the centre, and exhale as you twist to the other side.
- Repeat, coordinating breath with the movement.

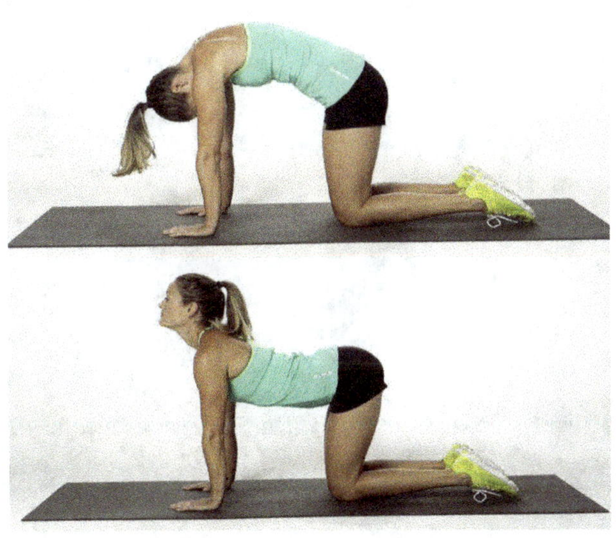

Somatic Cat-Cow Exploration:
- Start on your hands and knees in a tabletop position.
- Inhale, arching your back and lifting your tailbone (Cow).
- Exhale, rounding your spine and tucking your chin to your chest (Cat).
- Move between these positions slowly, focusing on the sensations in your core and spine.

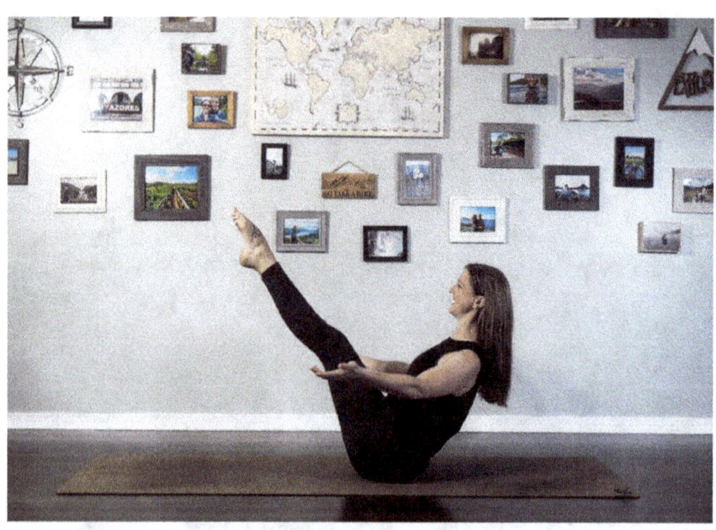

Intentional Boat Pose:
- Sit on the floor with your knees bent and feet flat.

- Inhale as you lift your legs, initiating the movement from your core.
- Exhale and engage your abdominal muscles to support the lifted position.
- Hold for a few breaths, maintaining awareness of the core, and lower down with control.

Approach these exercises with curiosity, allowing the experience to be a dialogue with your body. Through consistent practice, you not only strengthen your core but also deepen your connection with the intricate web of sensations within. In the chapters that follow, we will further explore core somatic exercises tailored to different fitness levels, ensuring that your journey into the power within is both accessible and transformative.

Chapter four

Release and Relaxation Techniques

As we delve deeper into the realm of somatic exercises, we encounter a sanctuary within—spaces and practices dedicated to the release of tension and the cultivation of profound relaxation. In this section, we will explore the essence of release and relaxation techniques, understanding how they become not only a respite from the demands of daily life but also a vital component in the holistic journey of self-discovery and well-being.

Progressive Muscle Relaxation for Stress Reduction:

Stress, that ubiquitous companion in the modern world, weaves its way into the fabric of our bodies, settling in muscles and tissues. In the pursuit of somatic well-being, we turn to a powerful ally—Progressive Muscle Relaxation (PMR). This technique, developed by physician Edmund Jacobson, involves systematically tensing and then releasing different muscle groups to induce a state of deep relaxation.

Begin with a comfortable seated or lying position. Let's consider the release of tension in the shoulders—a common repository for stress. Inhale as you consciously tense the muscles in your shoulders, raising them towards your ears. Hold the tension for a few seconds, and then exhale, allowing the shoulders to drop as you release the tension. Feel the warmth and lightness that follows, a tangible shift in the energy held within those muscles.

Extend this practice to other muscle groups—the neck, arms, back, and legs. With each intentional contraction and subsequent release, you create a symphony of relaxation that reverberates through your entire being. Progressive Muscle Relaxation becomes a rhythmic dance, a deliberate process of letting go that transcends the physical realm, extending into the corridors of mental and emotional release.

Somatic Exercises to Release Tension in Problem Areas:

Our bodies often bear the imprints of stress and daily wear in specific areas—perhaps the neck and shoulders from hours at a desk or the lower back from prolonged periods of sitting. Somatic exercises offer tailored solutions to release tension in these problem areas, providing a compassionate response to the body's call for relief.

Let's delve into a somatic exercise designed to release tension in the neck and shoulders. Begin by sitting comfortably, allowing your spine to elongate. Inhale deeply, and as you exhale, let your head tilt gently to one side, bringing your ear toward your shoulder. In this position, engage in a subtle rocking motion, exploring the range of motion and feeling the stretch along the side of your neck.

As you gradually introduce a gentle twist or nod, you encourage the release of tension that may have accumulated. This is not a forceful stretch but a mindful, explorative movement where you listen to the sensations in your neck and shoulders. With each breath, envision tension dissolving, making space for a renewed sense of ease.

Incorporating Mindfulness into Relaxation Practices:

Release and relaxation are not only physical phenomena but also states of mind. Mindfulness—the art of being present in the moment without judgement—becomes a companion in our journey toward relaxation. By infusing mindfulness into our relaxation practices, we deepen the connection between the body and mind, ushering in a sense of tranquillity that extends beyond the duration of the exercises.

Consider a simple mindfulness practice: deep belly breathing. As you inhale, allow your abdomen to expand, feeling the breath fill the lower lungs. Exhale slowly, feeling the gentle contraction of the abdominal muscles. In this rhythmic exchange, bring your attention to the sensations of the breath—the cool intake and warm release, the rise and fall of the belly. This focused awareness transforms breathing into a meditative act, grounding you in the present moment.

Extend this mindfulness to a full-body scan—a practice where you systematically bring awareness to each part of your body, starting from the toes and moving up to the crown of the head. As you scan, notice any areas of tension or discomfort without judgement. With each breath, invite those areas to soften and release. This mindful exploration becomes a self-inquiry, an intimate conversation with your body, and a pathway to holistic relaxation.

Examples of Release and Relaxation Techniques:

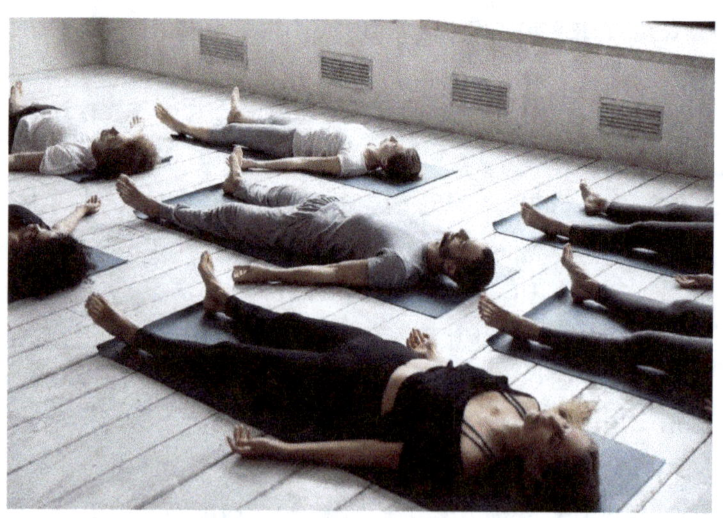

Progressive Muscle Relaxation (PMR):
- Find a comfortable position, either seated or lying down.

- Begin with your toes, inhaling as you tense the muscles, and exhaling as you release.
- Move systematically through different muscle groups—calves, thighs, abdomen, chest, shoulders, etc.
- Conclude with facial muscles and a full-body scan.
- Focus on the contrast between tension and relaxation in each muscle group.

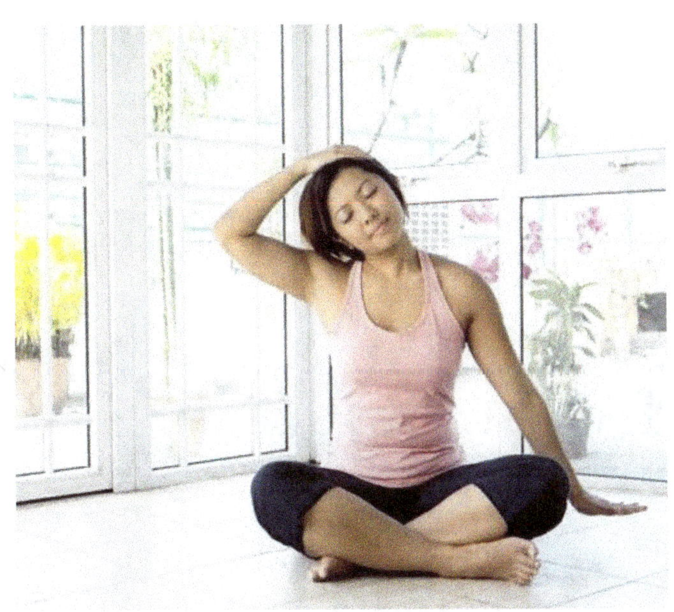

Neck and Shoulder Release Exercise:

- Sit comfortably with a straight spine.
- Inhale deeply, and as you exhale, tilt your head to one side, bringing your ear toward your shoulder.
- Engage in a gentle rocking motion, exploring the range of motion.
- Introduce subtle twists or nods, maintaining a sense of ease.
- Repeat on the other side, breathing deeply and releasing tension with each exhale.

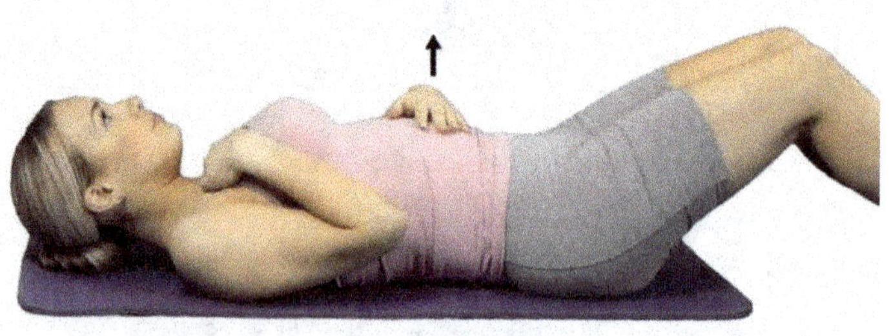

Mindful Belly Breathing:

- Find a comfortable seated or lying position.
- Inhale deeply, allowing your abdomen to expand.
- Exhale slowly, feeling the gentle contraction of the abdominal muscles.
- Focus your attention on the sensations of the breath—the rise and fall of the belly, the cool inhalation, and warm exhalation.
- Engage in this rhythmic breathing for several minutes, cultivating a sense of mindfulness and relaxation.

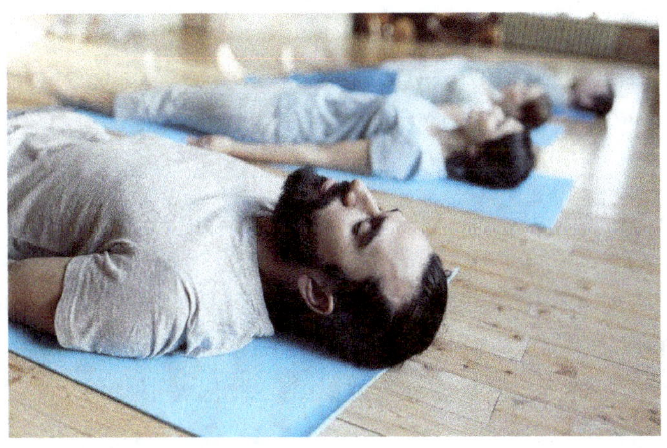

Full-Body Scan with Breath Awareness:
- Lie down in a comfortable position.
- Close your eyes and bring your awareness to your toes.
- Inhale deeply, and as you exhale, release any tension in your toes.
- Move systematically through each body part, from toes to head, incorporating deep breaths and intentional release.
- Notice and acknowledge any areas of tension without judgement, inviting them to soften with each breath.

These release and relaxation techniques are not just isolated practices; they are invitations to weave moments of tranquillity into the tapestry of your daily life. Through their regular incorporation, you create a sanctuary within, a space where tension dissipates, and the body-mind connection thrives. In the chapters that follow, we will continue to explore somatic exercises that nurture relaxation, ensuring that your journey is not just a series of exercises but a holistic embrace of well-being.

Chapter five

Somatic Movement Sequences

As we progress on our somatic journey, we encounter a realm of fluidity and grace—somatic movement sequences. In this section, we explore the essence of these sequences, understanding how they transcend the conventional boundaries of exercise, inviting us to dance with the wisdom inherent in our bodies. Join me as we unravel the transformative power of somatic movement, a symphony of mindful motion.

Full-Body Integration Exercises:

Somatic movement sequences, at their core, are invitations to orchestrate a dialogue between various parts of the body, fostering full-body integration. Unlike traditional workouts that may compartmentalise movements, somatic sequences encourage us to explore the connectivity between different regions, creating a harmonious flow of motion.

Consider a simple yet profound somatic movement: the spinal wave. In a standing position, start by initiating a gentle undulation from the base of the spine, allowing the movement to cascade through each vertebra. As you move upward, feel the engagement of abdominal muscles, the release of tension in the lower back, and the subtle opening of the chest. The spinal wave becomes a dance—a conversation between the various segments of your spine, fostering a sense of unity and coherence.

Extend this integration to include the arms and legs. Picture a sequence where the undulating motion of the spine seamlessly transitions into a graceful arm sweep and leg extension. Each movement informs the next, creating a continuous flow that engages the entire body. In these full-body integration exercises, we not only move with intention but also cultivate a heightened awareness of the interconnectedness that defines our physical being.

Dynamic Movements for Improved Flexibility:

Flexibility, a cornerstone of somatic well-being, is not just about achieving impressive stretches but embodying a suppleness that enhances our daily movements. Somatic movement sequences, designed with fluidity in mind, contribute to improved flexibility by encouraging dynamic, exploratory motions.

Let's delve into a dynamic sequence that enhances flexibility throughout the body—the somatic spiral. Begin in a seated position, and as you inhale, initiate a gentle twist to one side, allowing the movement to flow from the base of the spine to the crown of the head. Exhale as you return to the centre, and repeat on the other side. In this sequence, notice how the spine twists with ease, the shoulders open, and the entire torso engages in a rhythmic dance.

Now, integrate this somatic spiral with leg movements. As you twist to one side, extend the opposite leg, creating a diagonal stretch that extends from fingertips to toes. This dynamic sequence not only enhances flexibility in the spine but also explores the interconnectedness of the limbs. Each movement is an exploration, an opportunity to expand the range of motion and infuse flexibility into the very fabric of our being.

Sequences for Cardiovascular Health and Fat Burning:

While somatic practices often emphasise mindful and intentional movement, they can also contribute to cardiovascular health and fat burning through carefully crafted sequences. Somatic movement sequences for cardiovascular benefits prioritise fluid, continuous motion that elevates the heart rate without sacrificing the principles of mindfulness.

Picture a dynamic somatic sequence that combines rhythmic stepping with arm movements—a fusion of dance and exercise. Begin by stepping in place, feeling the connection between your feet and the ground. As you find your rhythm, introduce arm swings and circles, allowing the movements to synchronise with your breath. In this sequence, you engage in a cardiovascular workout that transcends the conventional notion of exercise—it becomes a celebration of movement.

Extend this sequence to include variations, such as side steps, forward and backward movements, and changes in arm patterns. The key is to maintain the fluidity and intentionality of the movements while elevating the heart rate. This somatic approach to cardiovascular health not only contributes to fat burning but also nurtures a joyful relationship with exercise—one that transcends the confines of traditional, rigid routines.

Examples of Somatic Movement Sequences:

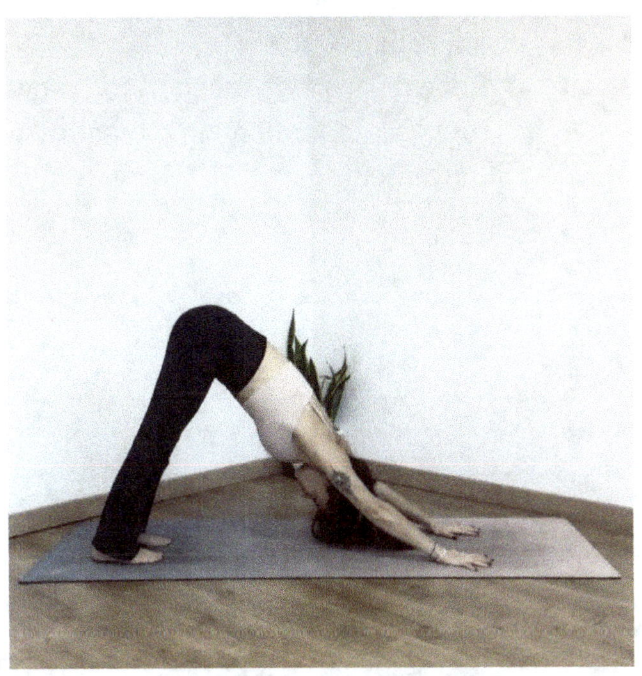

Spinal Wave Sequence:
- Stand with feet hip-width apart.

- Inhale and initiate a gentle forward tilt of the pelvis, allowing the wave to travel through the spine.
- Exhale as you sequentially engage each vertebra, creating a wave-like motion.
- Continue the wave as you arch the spine backward.
- Repeat the sequence for several rounds, coordinating breath with movement.

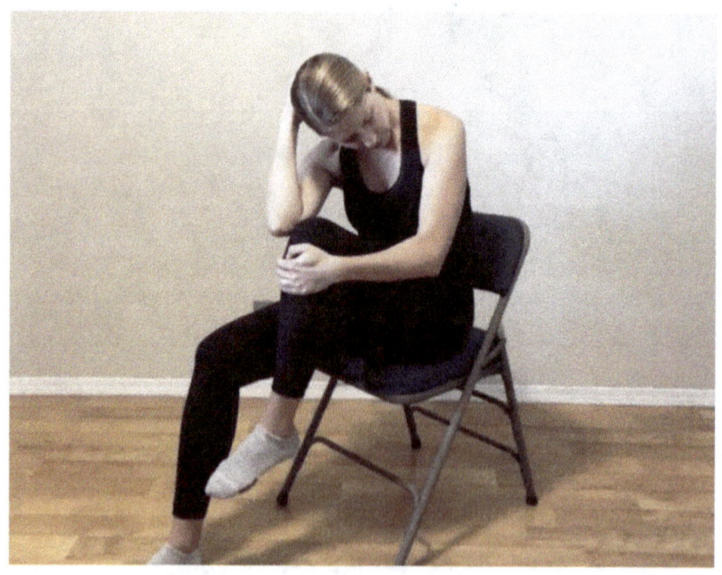

Somatic Spiral for Flexibility:
- Begin in a seated position with a straight spine.
- Inhale and twist to one side, allowing the movement to initiate from the base of the spine.
- Exhale and return to the centre.
- Repeat on the other side, exploring the range of motion in the spine.
- Integrate leg movements by extending the opposite leg during each twist.
- Flow between these movements, emphasising fluidity and exploration.

Cardiovascular Dance-Inspired Sequence:
- Start with rhythmic stepping in place.
- Introduce arm swings, circles, and variations in arm patterns.
- Explore side steps, forward and backward movements, and changes in pace.
- Maintain a continuous, fluid motion, synchronising movements with the breath.

- Let the sequence evolve into a dance-like expression of cardiovascular exercise.

Somatic movement sequences are invitations to engage in a mindful dance with our bodies. Through intentional, exploratory movements, we not only foster physical well-being but also cultivate a deeper connection with the inherent wisdom residing within. As we continue this journey, let these sequences be a celebration of the synergy between mind and body—a symphony of mindful motion that nourishes both the physical and the spiritual dimensions of our being.

Chapter six

Somatic Practices for Stress Reduction

In the hustle and bustle of our modern lives, stress has become an omnipresent force that not only affects our mental well-being but also plays a significant role in weight gain. In this chapter, we delve into the intricate relationship between stress and weight, explore somatic exercises designed to alleviate stress, and guide you in creating a personalised Somatic Stress Management Plan.

The Impact of Stress on Weight Gain

Stress, whether chronic or acute, triggers a cascade of physiological responses in the body, including the release of cortisol, often referred to as the "stress hormone." Elevated cortisol levels can contribute to weight gain, particularly around the abdominal area. This visceral fat accumulation is linked to various health issues, including cardiovascular diseases and metabolic disorders.

Chronic stress also influences our behaviours, leading to emotional eating and cravings for high-calorie comfort foods. These unhealthy eating patterns can further contribute to weight gain and hinder weight loss efforts.

To illustrate, imagine a scenario where work-related deadlines, family obligations, and financial pressures create a constant state of stress. In response, the body releases cortisol, prompting a heightened appetite for sugary and fatty foods. This can lead to overconsumption, disrupting the delicate balance of caloric intake and expenditure.

Somatic Exercises for Stress Relief

Somatic exercises offer a unique and effective approach to mitigate the impact of stress on both the body and mind. These exercises focus on releasing muscular tension, promoting body awareness, and restoring the natural flow of movement. Incorporating somatic practices into your routine can be transformative in reducing stress and its associated effects on weight.

Breathing Exercises for Stress Reduction:

Start with a simple seated or lying-down position. Inhale deeply through your nose, allowing your abdomen to expand, and exhale slowly through your mouth, releasing any tension. Focus on the rhythmic flow of your breath, engaging your diaphragm. This conscious breathing helps activate the parasympathetic nervous system, promoting relaxation.

Progressive Muscle Relaxation (PMR):

Lie down comfortably and systematically tense and then release each muscle group in your body, starting from your toes and working your way up to your head. This technique promotes awareness of tension and helps release stored stress in the muscles.

Mindful Movement Practices:

Engage in slow and deliberate movements, such as tai chi or gentle yoga. Pay close attention to each movement, allowing your mind to stay present and focused. These mindful practices not only enhance flexibility but also serve as moving meditations, reducing stress and anxiety.

Creating a Somatic Stress Management Plan

To harness the full potential of somatic exercises for stress reduction, it's essential to create a personalised Somatic Stress Management Plan. Tailoring your approach ensures that the plan aligns with your preferences, lifestyle, and stress triggers.

Identify Stress Triggers:

Begin by identifying the specific situations or circumstances that trigger stress in your life. Whether it's work-related pressures, relationship challenges, or external factors, understanding your stressors is the first step toward effective stress management.

Incorporate Daily Somatic Practices:

Integrate short somatic exercises into your daily routine. This could include dedicating a few minutes each morning to mindful breathing, practising PMR during breaks, or incorporating mindful movement into your exercise routine.

Consistency is key in reaping the long-term benefits of somatic stress reduction.

Create a Stress-Relief Toolkit:

Build a toolkit of somatic exercises that resonate with you. Experiment with different techniques and identify those that bring you the most relief. Your toolkit can include a variety of practices, allowing flexibility in addressing stress based on your current needs and circumstances.

Establish Mindful Eating Habits:

Recognize the connection between stress and eating habits. Develop mindful eating practices, such as savouring each bite, listening to your body's hunger and fullness cues, and choosing nourishing foods. This mindful approach to eating can break the cycle of stress-induced overeating.

Seek Professional Guidance if Needed:

If stress is significantly impacting your life, consider seeking guidance from a somatic therapist, mindfulness coach, or mental health professional. They can provide personalised strategies and support to address the root causes of stress and guide you in implementing effective somatic practices.

Chapter seven

Personalising Your Somatic Weight Loss Journey

In the pursuit of weight loss, recognizing that each individual is unique in their needs, goals, and fitness levels is paramount. This chapter delves into the process of personalising your somatic weight loss journey, guiding you through the essential steps of assessing your needs, adapting exercises to your fitness level, and seamlessly incorporating somatic practices into your daily life.

Assessing Individual Needs and Goals

Understanding your body and setting realistic goals are crucial steps in any weight loss journey. Somatic exercises, rooted in mind-body connection, require a personalised approach. Begin by taking stock of your current physical condition, identifying any areas of discomfort, and pinpointing your specific weight loss objectives.

Example:

Jane, a 35-year-old office worker, identifies chronic lower back pain and stress-related eating as her primary concerns. Her goal is not just shedding pounds but cultivating a healthier relationship with her body.

To assess your needs and goals effectively, consider the following:

Physical Assessment:
- Evaluate your current fitness level, flexibility, and strength.
- Identify areas of tension or pain.
- Reflect on your daily activities that may impact your body.

Emotional and Psychological Assessment:
- Recognize emotional triggers related to eating habits.
- Assess stress levels and how they manifest in your body.
- Clarify your motivations and attitudes toward weight loss.

Setting Realistic Goals:
- Establish short-term and long-term objectives.

- Ensure your goals align with your lifestyle and commitments.
- Prioritise health and well-being over arbitrary numbers on a scale.

Adapting Somatic Exercises to Fitness Levels

Somatic exercises are designed to be gentle and accessible, making them suitable for individuals of varying fitness levels. Adapting these exercises to your personal capabilities ensures a safe and effective practice that promotes gradual progress.

Example:

John, a 50-year-old with limited mobility due to a previous injury, wants to integrate somatic exercises into his routine. He starts with modified movements and progresses at a pace that suits his body.

To adapt somatic exercises to your fitness level:

Start with Basic Movements:
- Initiate your practice with foundational exercises.

- Focus on awareness and precision before intensity.

Modify Poses as Needed:

- Adjust movements to accommodate limitations or discomfort.
- Use props or support to enhance stability.

Gradual Progression:

- Increase the complexity of exercises as your body adapts.
- Listen to your body and avoid pushing beyond your comfort zone.

Incorporating Somatics into Daily Life

For sustainable weight loss, somatic practices should seamlessly integrate into your daily routine. Consistency is key, and incorporating these exercises into your lifestyle fosters lasting benefits.

Example:

Lily, a busy mother of two, incorporates short somatic exercises into her daily routine, finding moments of tranquillity amidst her hectic schedule.

To incorporate somatic practices into daily life:

Create a Routine:
- Designate specific times for somatic exercises.
- Integrate them into existing routines, like morning or bedtime rituals.

Mindful Movement Breaks:
- Take short breaks during the day for gentle stretches or breathing exercises.
- Use somatic practices as a tool to alleviate stress during work hours.

Mindful Eating Practices:
- Apply somatic principles to your meals, practising mindful eating.
- Pay attention to hunger and fullness cues, savouring each bite.

Family Involvement:
- Encourage family or friends to join, making somatic exercises a shared activity.
- Create a supportive environment that fosters healthy habits.

personalising your somatic weight loss journey is a holistic approach that acknowledges the uniqueness of your body and circumstances. By assessing your needs, adapting exercises to your fitness level, and incorporating somatic practices into your daily life, you pave the way for sustainable and meaningful transformation. Remember, this is not just a journey to lose weight but a voyage towards greater self-awareness, well-being, and a harmonious relationship with your body.

<u>Chapter eight</u>

<u>Maintaining Progress and Long-Term Success</u>

Strategies for Sustainable Weight Management

Sustainable weight management involves adopting habits that can be maintained over a lifetime. Diets that promise quick fixes often lead to short-term results, and individuals find themselves trapped in a cycle of weight loss and gain. Somatic exercises offer a holistic approach to sustainable weight management by addressing both the physical and mental aspects of wellness.

Understanding Nutritional Balance: One crucial aspect of sustainable weight management is cultivating a balanced approach to nutrition. Somatic practices encourage mindful eating, fostering a deeper connection with the body's hunger and fullness cues. Incorporating nutrient-dense foods, such as fruits, vegetables, lean proteins, and whole grains, into your diet can provide the energy needed for somatic exercises while supporting overall health.

Hydration and Body Awareness: Staying well-hydrated is vital for overall health and weight management. Somatic exercises emphasise body awareness, encouraging individuals to listen to their bodies' signals, including thirst. Maintaining proper hydration levels supports optimal bodily functions and can contribute to better exercise performance.

Consistency Over Perfection: Sustainable weight management is not about perfection but rather consistency. Small, consistent changes in both exercise routines and dietary habits can lead to lasting results. Somatic exercises, being gentle and adaptable, can be incorporated into daily life, making it easier to maintain consistency without the risk of burnout.

Building a Consistent Somatic Exercise Routine

Consistency is the cornerstone of any successful fitness journey. Establishing and maintaining a regular somatic exercise routine not only contributes to physical well-being but also nurtures a positive relationship between the mind and body.

Setting Realistic Goals: When building a somatic exercise routine, it's essential to set realistic and achievable goals. Start with manageable time commitments and gradually increase intensity as your body becomes more accustomed to the exercises. Somatic practices prioritise quality over quantity, ensuring that each movement is performed with mindfulness and intention.

Integrating Somatic Exercises into Daily Life: Somatic exercises need not be confined to a specific workout session. Infusing somatic movements into daily activities, such as incorporating mindful stretches during breaks or practising deep breathing while commuting, ensures a consistent engagement with the mind-body connection. This integration makes somatic practices more sustainable in the long run.

Variety and Adaptability: To maintain interest and motivation, incorporate a variety of somatic exercises into your routine. This not only challenges different muscle groups but also prevents monotony. The adaptability of somatic practices allows individuals to modify routines based on their energy levels, ensuring a consistent yet flexible approach to exercise.

Celebrating Achievements and Staying Motivated

Celebrating achievements, whether big or small, plays a crucial role in staying motivated on the path to long-term success. Acknowledging progress fosters a positive mindset and reinforces the commitment to the weight loss journey.

Tracking Progress: Keeping a journal to track somatic exercise routines, dietary choices, and overall well-being provides a tangible record of progress. Reflecting on achievements, such as increased flexibility, enhanced body awareness, or weight loss milestones, serves as a powerful motivator to continue the journey.

Positive Reinforcement: Positive reinforcement is a fundamental aspect of staying motivated. Rewarding yourself for achieving goals, be it with a small treat, a relaxing day, or the acknowledgment of a job well done, reinforces the positive behaviours associated with somatic exercises and healthy lifestyle choices.

Community Support: Sharing achievements with a supportive community can provide an additional layer of motivation. Online forums, local groups, or workout buddies create a sense of accountability and encouragement. Celebrating milestones collectively can make the weight loss journey more enjoyable and less isolating.

Mind-Body Connection: Recognizing and celebrating achievements goes beyond physical changes. Embracing the enhanced mind-body connection that somatic practices cultivate is an achievement in itself. Celebrate the moments of mindfulness, the deeper understanding of your body, and the overall improvement in well-being.

28 DAYS CHALLENGE

Embarking on this 28-day journey of somatic exercises for weight loss is a commendable step towards enhancing both your physical and emotional well-being. As you commit to this challenge, remember that every small effort contributes to significant progress.

Encourage yourself daily, celebrate your achievements, and be patient with the process. Consistency is key, so embrace the routines with dedication. Begin each day with a positive mindset, acknowledging that these exercises are not just about shedding pounds but also fostering flexibility, strength, and balance.

Listen to your body; it's your guide through this transformative experience. If you encounter challenges, modify the exercises to suit your comfort level. Feel free to explore and personalise the routines to make them enjoyable.

Stay connected with a community or share your progress with friends and family. Support can make a significant difference in staying motivated.

Embrace the journey, relish the changes, and savour the improvements in both your physical and emotional well-being.

You've got this! Here's to a healthier, happier you.

day	Morning routine	Mid-day break	Afternoon energizer	Evening relaxation	tick
1	Seated body scan	Neck and Shoulder Rolls	Standing Forward Fold	Mindful breathing	
2	Pelvic tilts	Wrist and ankle circles	Cat-cow stretch	Body scan with deep relaxation	
3	Diaphragmatic Breathing	Seated twist	Leg swings	Progressive Muscle Relaxation	
4	Seated forward bend	Side body stretch	Gentle spinal twist	Mindful walking meditation	
5	Pelvic clocks	Seated desk stretch	Seated hamstring stretch	Relaxing shoulder opener	
6	Full body scan	Dynamic arm swings	Seated hip opener	Guided meditation for sleep	
7	Seated spinal twist	Ankle rolls and flexes	Standing calf raises	Body scan with breath awareness	
8	Somatic	Neck	Forward	Mindful	

	squats	nods and turns	fold with arm reach	breath and stretch	
9	Shoulder rolls and shrugs	Seated side stretch	Hip circles	Progressive relaxation	
10	Seated cat-cow stretch	Chest opener	Seated leg extension	Evening body scan	
11	Pelvic figure-eight movements	Seated shoulder opener	Standing hip flexor stretch	Mindful yoga nidra	
12	Mindful breathing and lift arms	Seated forward fold with rotation	Gentle leg swings	Deep relaxation with visualisation	
13	Seated pelvic tilts	Wrist and ankle flexibility	Gentle neck stretches	Breath awareness meditation	
14	Somatic walking meditation	Seated spinal twist and side bend	Standing calf stretch	Full body relaxation	
15	Seated hip hinge	Arm circles and shoulder rolls	Side-lying leg lifts	Guided body scan with breath	
16	Seated Diaphragmatic	Neck Stretches	Forward Fold with Leg Cross	Mindful Evening Stretches	

	Breathing				
17	Seated Twist and Reach	Seated Desk Stretches	Dynamic Ankle Rolls	Relaxing Breath and Stretch	
18	Somatic Yoga Sequence	Wrist and Finger Exercises	Standing Side Bend	Body Scan for Tension Release	
19	Seated Shoulder and Arm Stretch	Pelvic Tilts with Arm Movement	Leg Swings with Arm Circles	Evening Mindful Movement	
20	Seated Forward Bend with Rotation	Ankle Circles and Point Flexes	Seated Hip Circles	Deep Breathing and Stretch	
21	Neck Nods and Tilts	Seated Side Stretch with Reach	Standing Forward Fold with Twist	Mindful Relaxation Techniques	
22	Seated Pelvic Clocks	Dynamic Arm Swings	Gentle Seated Twists	Guided Progressive Relaxation	
23	Somatic Squats with Breath	Neck and Shoulder Stretches	Standing Calf Raises	Evening Yoga Nidra	
24	Seated Cat-Cow Stretch	Wrist and Ankle Circles	Forward Fold with Arm Reach	Mindful Breath and Stretch	

25	Pelvic Figure-Eight Movements	Seated Forward Fold with Rotation	Standing Hip Flexor Stretch	Body Scan with Visualization	
26	Shoulder Rolls and Shrugs	Seated Hip Opener	Gentle Leg Swings	Deep Relaxation with Breath	
27	Seated Spinal Twist with Side Bend	Chest Opener	Seated Leg Extension	Evening Mindful Body Scan	
28	Full Body Scan and Stretch	Relaxing Shoulder Opener	Mindful Walking Meditation	Closing Meditation	

I recommend the book "Wall Pilates for Women" by Angel Rosie to all women interested in exploring the benefits of wall pilates. This comprehensive guide provides insightful and accessible routines specifically tailored for women, incorporating the support of a wall to enhance the effectiveness of Pilates exercises.

Angel Rosie's expertise shines through in her approach, making the exercises not only effective for toning and strengthening but also enjoyable. Whether you're a beginner or experienced in Pilates, this book offers a progressive and customizable program to suit various fitness levels.

Dive into "Wall Pilates for Women" to discover how this innovative approach can transform your fitness journey. With clear instructions and illustrations, Angel Rosie empowers women to embrace the power of Pilates, utilising the support of a wall to achieve optimal results. Enhance your strength, flexibility, and overall well-being with this empowering resource.

We hope you find the 28-day somatic exercises for weight loss in this book transformative and enriching. As you embark on this journey, we encourage you to share your experiences and the positive changes you've noticed.

Your feedback is invaluable, not only for us but for fellow readers seeking inspiration. If this book has contributed to your well-being, kindly consider leaving a review. Share your insights, progress, and any tips you've discovered along the way.

Your review could be the motivation someone else needs to take the first step towards a healthier lifestyle. We appreciate your time and commitment to this transformative process.

Thank you for being part of this journey.

____

____

____

____

____

____

<u>TESTIMONIALS</u>

TESTIMONIALS

www.ingramcontent.com/pod-product-compliance
Lightning Source LLC
Chambersburg PA
CBHW050849260726
48660CB00006B/2528